RENAL DIET COOKBOOK FOR BEGINNERS

Simple and easy way to ignite your journey of kidney health with low potassium, low sodium and low phosphorus delicious recipe

Avila Wanda

Table of contents

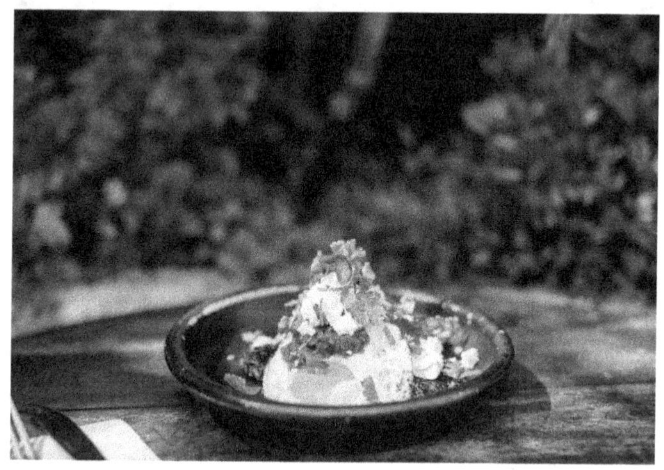

Introduction

In the bustling realm of modern nutrition, where health-conscious individuals seek optimal well-being, the Renal Diet emerges as a crucial player in supporting kidney health. Introducing the *"Renal Diet Cookbook for Beginners,"* a culinary guide designed to transform dietary choices into a journey of delicious, kidney-friendly meals.

Navigating the delicate balance of flavors and nutrients, this cookbook is crafted with the understanding that individuals with renal concerns require a specialized approach to nutrition. The introductory chapters unravel the mysteries of the renal diet, providing readers with a comprehensive understanding of the essential elements that define kidney-friendly eating. From controlling sodium intake to managing phosphorus levels, the cookbook establishes a solid foundation for maintaining renal health.

What sets this cookbook apart is its dedication to simplicity and accessibility. The recipes within are thoughtfully curated for beginners, ensuring that even those with limited culinary expertise can embark on this gastronomic adventure with confidence. Each recipe is a harmonious blend of wholesome ingredients, carefully selected to cater to the unique nutritional needs of individuals with compromised kidney function.

Beyond the realm of nourishment, the "Renal Diet Cookbook for Beginners" transcends into a culinary companion that inspires and empowers. It goes beyond mere sustenance, transforming meals into a celebration of health and vitality. With a focus on diverse, flavorful dishes, this cookbook aims to prove that adhering to a renal diet doesn't mean compromising on taste.

Whether you are embarking on a renal diet journey for the first time or seeking fresh inspiration to revitalize your culinary repertoire, this cookbook beckons you into a world where vibrant flavors and kidney health unite. Embrace the art of nourishing your body with the "Renal Diet Cookbook for Beginners" – a delightful compass guiding you towards a path of well-being, one delectable recipe at a time.

Chapter one

What is renal diet

A renal diet, also known as a kidney-friendly diet, is a specialized eating plan designed to promote kidney health and manage conditions such as chronic kidney disease (CKD). The primary goals of a renal diet are to reduce the workload on the kidneys, maintain a balance of essential nutrients, and manage fluid and electrolyte levels.

Key components of a renal diet include:

1. **Controlled Protein Intake:** Limiting high-protein foods to reduce the strain on the kidneys and minimize the production of waste products.

2. **Sodium Restriction:** Managing sodium intake to help control blood pressure and fluid balance, as excessive sodium can contribute to fluid retention.

3. **Phosphorus Management:** Monitoring phosphorus intake, as impaired kidneys may struggle to

regulate phosphorus levels, leading to bone and cardiovascular issues.

4. **Potassium Regulation:** Adjusting potassium intake, as kidneys with reduced function may struggle to eliminate excess potassium, which can affect heart health.

5. **Fluid Control:** Monitoring fluid intake to prevent fluid overload, a common concern in kidney disease that can lead to swelling and high blood pressure.

6. **Calorie Adjustment:** Modifying caloric intake based on individual needs, as CKD can affect

metabolism and energy requirements.

The *"Renal Diet Cookbook for Beginners"* would likely offer recipes that adhere to these dietary principles, providing flavorful and nutritious options while respecting the limitations imposed by kidney-related health concerns. Always consult with a healthcare professional or a registered dietitian to personalize dietary recommendations based on individual health conditions and needs.

Chapter two

Benefits of renal diet

The renal diet offers several benefits for individuals with kidney-related health concerns, particularly those with conditions like chronic kidney disease (CKD). Here are some key benefits:

1. **Slow Progression of Kidney Disease:** A renal diet, by controlling protein intake and managing other nutrients, aims to slow down the progression of kidney disease. This can help

preserve kidney function over time.

2. **Blood Pressure Management:** Sodium restriction in a renal diet helps control blood pressure, a critical aspect of kidney health. Managing blood pressure is essential for preventing further damage to the kidneys.

3. **Fluid Balance:** The renal diet includes guidelines for managing fluid intake, helping to prevent fluid retention and maintain a healthy fluid balance in the body.

4. **Electrolyte Control:** By regulating potassium and phosphorus intake, the renal diet helps prevent

imbalances in electrolytes. This is crucial for avoiding complications such as abnormal heart rhythms and bone disorders.

5. **Nutritional Support:** Despite restrictions, a well-balanced renal diet ensures that individuals receive essential nutrients. This helps prevent malnutrition and supports overall health.

6. **Symptom Management:** Following a renal diet can alleviate symptoms associated with kidney disease, such as fatigue, nausea, and swelling. By addressing nutritional imbalances, individuals

may experience an improvement in their overall well-being.

7. **Cardiovascular Health:** The renal diet's emphasis on controlling blood pressure and managing other cardiovascular risk factors indirectly benefits heart health, reducing the risk of cardiovascular complications often associated with kidney disease.

8. **Improved Quality of Life:** Adhering to a renal diet with carefully crafted, flavorful recipes can make the dietary restrictions more manageable and enjoyable. This can contribute to an improved

quality of life for individuals with kidney-related health concerns.

It's crucial for individuals to work closely with healthcare professionals and registered dietitians to tailor the renal diet to their specific needs, ensuring optimal nutritional support while managing kidney-related conditions.

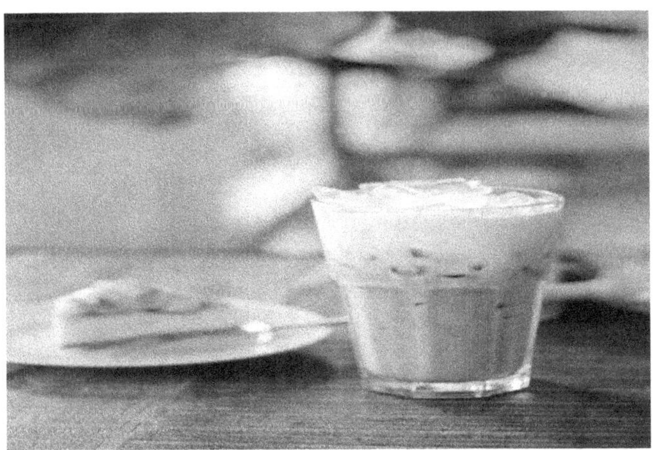

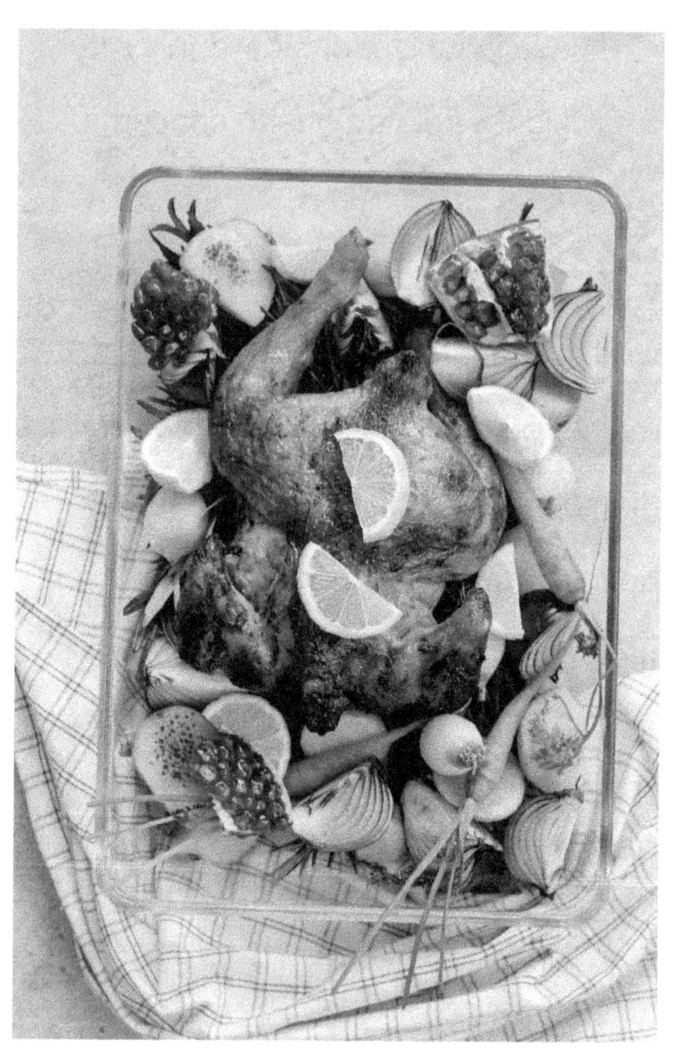

Chapter three

Specific Nutritional recommendation

Specific nutritional recommendations for a renal diet may vary based on an individual's health status, stage of kidney disease, and other medical conditions. However, here are some general guidelines commonly associated with a renal diet:

1. **Protein Intake:**

   - Eat fewer meals heavy in protein to lessen the strain on your kidneys.

o Choose high-quality protein
sources such as lean meats,
poultry, fish, eggs, and dairy
in moderation.

o Adjust protein intake based
on the stage of kidney
disease.

2. **Sodium (Salt) Restriction:**

o To assist control blood
pressure and fluid balance,
reduce your consumption of
salt.

o Avoid processed and
high-sodium foods.

o Instead of using salt to flavor
food, use herbs and spices.

3. Phosphorus Control:

- Monitor phosphorus intake, as impaired kidneys may have difficulty regulating phosphorus levels.
- Limit consumption of phosphorus-rich foods like dairy products, nuts, and seeds.

4. Potassium Regulation:

- Adjust potassium intake based on blood levels and kidney function.
- Limit high-potassium foods like bananas, oranges, tomatoes, and potatoes.

5. **Fluid Management:**

- Control fluid intake to
   prevent fluid overload.

- Monitor thirst and choose
   foods with lower fluid
   content.

6. **Caloric Adjustment:**

- Adjust caloric intake based
   on individual needs,
   considering factors like age,
   weight, and activity level.

- Ensure an adequate intake
   of calories to prevent
   malnutrition.

7. **Vitamins and Minerals:**

- Supplement vitamins and
   minerals if there is a

deficiency due to dietary
restrictions.

- Vitamin D and calcium
  supplements may be
  necessary to support bone
  health.

8. **Monitoring Blood Pressure and Blood Sugar:**

- Check your blood sugar and
  blood pressure on a regular
  basis.
- Manage diabetes if present,
  as it can impact kidney
  health.

It's crucial for individuals to work closely with healthcare professionals, including registered dietitians, to tailor these recommendations to their specific circumstances. Regular monitoring and adjustments to the renal diet can help manage kidney-related conditions effectively.

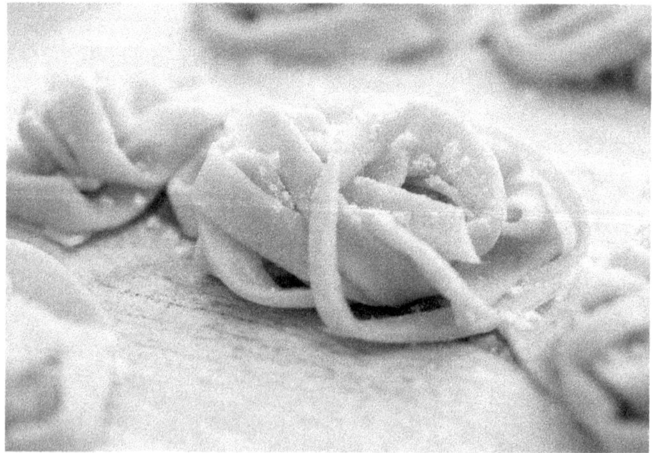

Chapter four

List of foods to limits or avoid

Individuals following a renal diet, especially those with kidney disease, are often advised to limit or avoid certain foods to manage their condition effectively. Here's a list of foods that are typically restricted in a renal diet:

1. **High-Protein Foods:**
   - Red meat (beef, lamb, pork)
   - Processed meats (sausages, hot dogs, bacon)
   - Organ meats (liver, kidneys)
2. **High-Sodium Foods:**

- Processed and packaged
  foods

- Canned soups and broths

- Deli meats and cured meats

- Salted snacks (chips,
  pretzels)

3. **High-Phosphorus Foods:**

- Dairy products (milk,
  cheese, yogurt)

- Nuts and seeds

- Chocolate and cocoa
  products

- Colas and dark sodas

4. **High-Potassium Foods:**

- Bananas

- Oranges and orange juice

- Tomatoes and tomato

  products

- Potatoes and sweet

  potatoes

5. High-Fluid Foods:

- Water-rich fruits

  (watermelon, cantaloupe)

- Soups with high liquid

  content

- Ice cream and gelatin

6. Certain Vegetables:

- Spinach and Swiss chard

  (high in potassium)

- Beets (contain both

  potassium and phosphorus)

- Tomatoes (contain

  potassium)

7. **Salt and Sodium-Containing Condiments:**

    - Soy sauce and other salty condiments

    - Bouillon cubes and powders

8. **Processed Convenience Foods:**

    - Instant noodles and packaged meals

    - Frozen dinners and pre-packaged snacks

9. **Alcohol:**

    - Limit alcohol intake, as it can contribute to dehydration and affect kidney function.

It's important to note that individual dietary recommendations may vary based on factors such as the stage of kidney disease and other health conditions. Always seek the counsel of a licensed dietician or healthcare expert for individualized recommendations and direction tailored to your unique requirements.

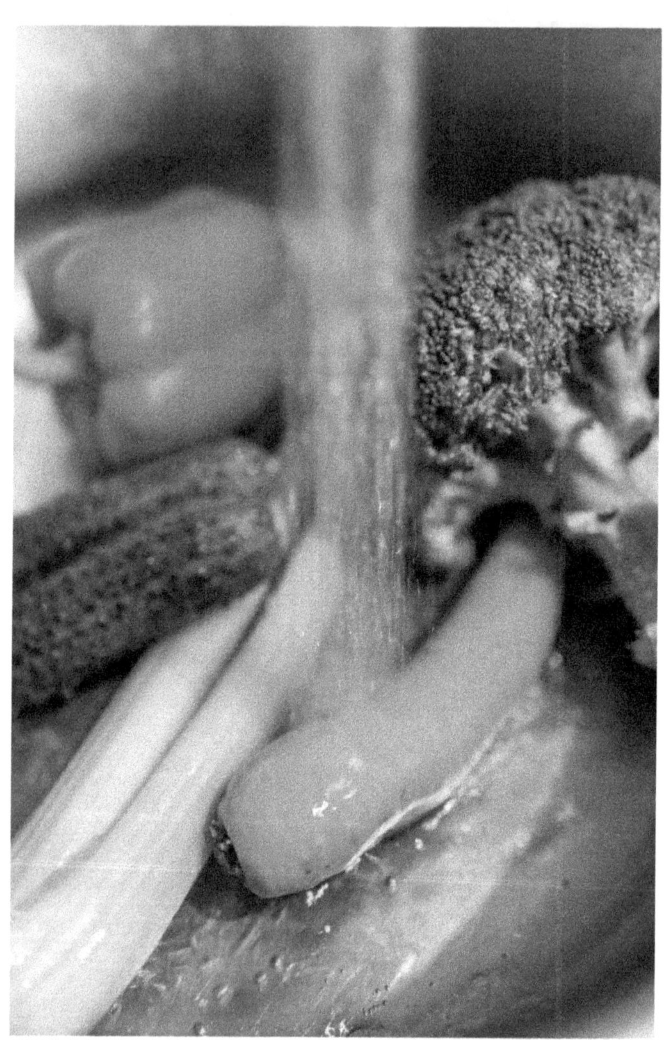

Chapter five

Shopping list

Creating a renal-friendly shopping list is essential for individuals following a renal diet. Here's a sample shopping list that focuses on nutrient-rich, kidney-friendly foods:

Proteins:

1. Lean cuts of poultry (chicken or turkey breast)
2. Fresh fish (salmon, tilapia, cod)
3. Eggs

4. dairy goods low in fat (in moderation, milk, yogurt, and cheese)

Vegetables:

5. Leafy greens with lower potassium content (lettuce, cabbage, kale)

6. Cauliflower and broccoli
7. Bell peppers
8. Green beans

Fruits:

9. Apples

10.   Berries (strawberries,
       blueberries, raspberries)
11.   Pineapple
12.   Peaches

Grains and Starches:

13. White rice

14.   White bread or whole grain
       bread in moderation
15.   Pasta (choose varieties with
       lower phosphorus content)

Snacks:

16. Unsalted popcorn

17.   Rice cakes

18.   Homemade trail mix with kidney-friendly nuts (almonds, cashews)

Dairy Alternatives:

19. Rice milk or almond milk (choose low-phosphorus options)

Beverages:

20. Water

21.   Herbal teas (caffeine-free)

22.   Freshly squeezed fruit juices in moderation

Condiments:

23. Fresh herbs and spices for flavoring (parsley, basil, oregano)

24. Olive oil
25. Low-sodium salad dressings

Desserts (in moderation):

26. Sorbet

27. Angel food cake

Miscellaneous:

28. Unsalted butter

29.   Cooking oils (olive oil, canola oil)

30.   Canned vegetables with low sodium content (rinse before use)

For information on potassium, phosphorus, and salt contents, always read food labels. Consider consulting with a registered dietitian for personalized guidance and adjustments based on your specific dietary needs and health status. Regularly updating your shopping list ensures you have a variety of kidney-friendly options to create balanced and flavorful meals.

Chapter six

Breakfast recipes

A renal diet cookbook for beginners can offer a variety of nutritious and kidney-friendly breakfast options. Consider including recipes like:

1. **Quinoa Breakfast Bowl:**
   - Cooked quinoa as a base.
   - Add diced fruits like apples or berries.
   - For extra crunch, put chopped nuts on top.
2. **Vegetable Omelet:**

- Whisk together egg whites and pour into a non-stick pan.
- Fill with kidney-friendly vegetables like bell peppers, spinach, and tomatoes.

3. **Sweet Potato Hash:**

- Dice sweet potatoes and sauté with onions and bell peppers.
- For taste, add herbs like rosemary and thyme to the dish.

4. **Greek Yogurt Parfait:**

- Layer low-phosphorus Greek yogurt with sliced bananas or peaches.

- Sprinkle with a handful of low-potassium granola.

5. Millet Porridge:

- Cook millet in almond milk until creamy.

- Add a touch of cinnamon and sliced strawberries for sweetness.

6. Avocado Toast on Whole Grain Bread:

- Spread mashed avocado on whole grain toast.

- Sprinkle it with sesame seeds and a dash of lemon juice.

Remember to limit sodium and phosphorus content in these recipes, and consult with a healthcare professional for personalized dietary advice.

Recipes for lunch

Certainly! Here are a few renal-friendly lunch recipes for beginners:

1. **Grilled Chicken Salad:**
   - Grilled chicken breast strips on a bed of mixed greens.

- Add cherry tomatoes,
    cucumber slices, and a
    sprinkle of feta cheese.
  - Dress with a low-sodium
    vinaigrette.

2. **Salmon and Quinoa Bowl:**
  - Baked salmon fillet served
    over a bed of cooked
    quinoa.
  - Add steamed asparagus and
    drizzle with a lemon-dill
    sauce.

3. **Vegetarian Stir-Fry:**
  - Stir-fry kidney-friendly
    vegetables like bell peppers,
    broccoli, and snap peas.

- Add tofu cubes for protein
    and flavor.

  - Serve over brown rice.

4. **Turkey and Vegetable Wrap:**

  - Whole-grain wrap filled with
    lean turkey slices.

  - Add shredded lettuce, diced
    tomatoes, and a smear of
    low-sodium hummus.

5. **Eggplant Parmesan:**

  - Baked slices of eggplant
    layered with low-sodium
    tomato sauce and
    mozzarella.

  - Serve over whole-grain
    pasta or with a side of
    steamed vegetables.

6. **Lentil Soup:**

   - Hearty lentil soup with carrots, celery, and low-sodium vegetable broth.
   - Season with herbs like cumin and coriander for extra flavor.

Remember to control sodium and phosphorus intake, and tailor portion sizes based on individual dietary needs. Always consult with a healthcare professional for personalized dietary guidance.

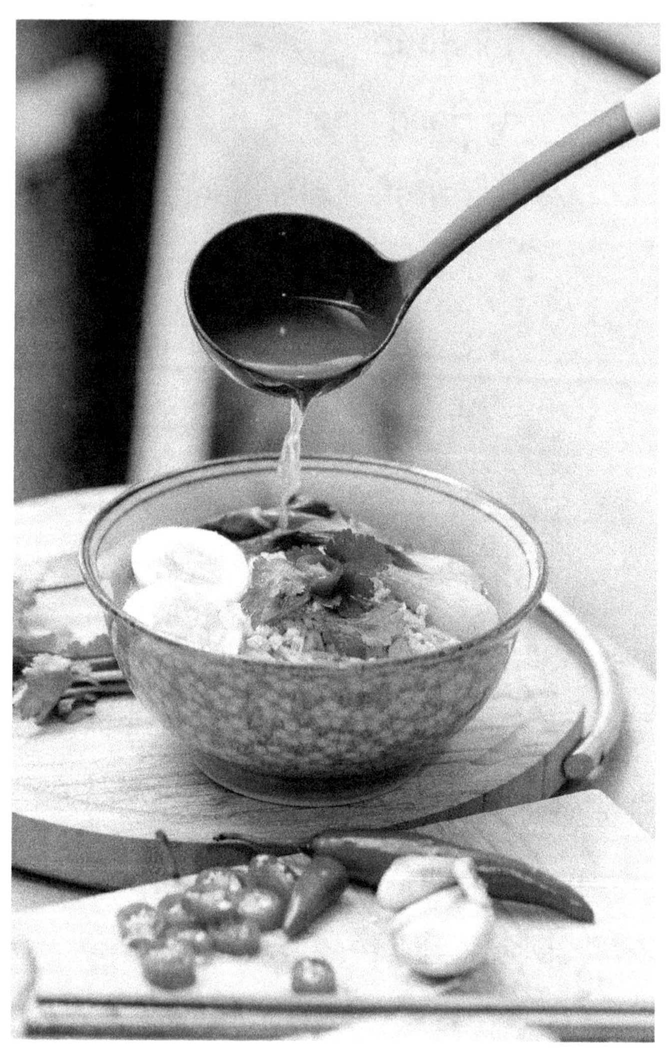

Chapter seven

Recipes for dinner

Certainly! Here's an extensive collection of renal-friendly dinner recipes for beginners:

1. **Baked Lemon Herb Chicken:**
   - Marinate chicken breasts with lemon juice, garlic, and herbs.
   - Bake until golden brown and serve with roasted sweet potatoes and steamed green beans.

2. **Shrimp and Vegetable Skewers:**

- Thread shrimp, cherry tomatoes, and zucchini onto skewers.
- Grill or broil until the shrimp are cooked through. Serve with a side of quinoa.

3. **Mushroom and Spinach Stuffed Peppers:**

- Mix sautéed mushrooms and spinach with cooked brown rice.
- After stuffing the mixture into the bell peppers, bake them until they are soft.

4. **Chickpea and Spinach Curry:**

- Simmer chickpeas, spinach, and diced tomatoes in a

coconut milk-based curry
sauce.

  ○ Serve over basmati rice or
    quinoa.

5. **Baked Cod with Herb Crust:**

  ○ Coat cod filets with a mixture
    of breadcrumbs, parsley,
    and lemon zest.

  ○ Bake until the fish flakes
    easily. Pair with roasted
    Brussels sprouts.

6. **Vegetable and Lentil Stew:**

  ○ Combine lentils, carrots,
    celery, and low-sodium
    vegetable broth in a slow
    cooker.

- Season with cumin and
  coriander, and cook until
  lentils are tender.

7. **Turkey and Vegetable Stir-Fry:**

   - Stir-fry lean ground turkey
     with kidney-friendly
     vegetables like bell peppers
     and broccoli.

   - Season with low-sodium soy
     sauce and serve over brown
     rice.

8. **Egg Fried Rice with Vegetables:**

   - Sauté mixed vegetables like
     peas, carrots, and bell
     peppers in a pan.

   - Stir in cooked brown rice
     and scrambled eggs,

seasoning with low-sodium
soy sauce.

9. Grilled Portobello Mushrooms with Balsamic Glaze:

- Marinate portobello mushrooms in balsamic vinegar and olive oil.
- Grill until tender and drizzle with a reduced balsamic glaze. Serve with a side salad.

10. Baked Turkey Meatballs:

- Combine ground turkey with breadcrumbs, egg whites, and Italian herbs.
- Bake meatballs and serve with a low-phosphorus

tomato sauce over whole-grain pasta.

Remember to adapt recipes based on individual dietary restrictions, and consult with a healthcare professional for personalized advice. Adjusting portion sizes and monitoring phosphorus and sodium content is crucial for those following a renal diet.

Chapter eight

Recipes for snacks

Certainly! Here are some kidney-friendly snack ideas for beginners:

1. **Hummus and Veggie Sticks:**
   - Dip cucumber, carrot, and bell pepper sticks into low-sodium hummus.

2. **Fresh Fruit Salad:**
   - Mix together diced watermelon, strawberries, and pineapple for a refreshing fruit salad.

3. **Greek Yogurt with Berries:**

- Enjoy a bowl of low-phosphorus Greek yogurt topped with fresh berries.

4. **Rice Cake with Almond Butter:**

   - Spread almond butter on a rice cake for a satisfying and kidney-friendly snack.

5. **Hard-Boiled Eggs:**

   - Hard boil eggs and sprinkle with a pinch of salt or herbs for added flavor.

6. **Nuts and Seeds Mix:**

   - Combine kidney-friendly nuts like almonds and seeds like pumpkin seeds for a crunchy snack.

7. **Apple Slices with Cinnamon:**

   - Slice apples and sprinkle with a dash of cinnamon for a sweet and nutritious snack.

8. **Cottage Cheese with Pineapple:**

   - Pair low-sodium cottage cheese with diced pineapple for a protein-packed snack.

9. **Vegetable Salsa with Baked Tortilla Chips:**

   - Mix diced tomatoes, onions, and cilantro for a fresh salsa. Serve with baked tortilla chips.

10. **Roasted Chickpeas:**

- Toss chickpeas with olive oil and your favorite spices, then roast until crunchy.

Remember to monitor portion sizes and choose snacks that fit within individual dietary guidelines. It's essential to consult with a healthcare professional or dietitian for personalized advice based on specific health needs.

Chapter nine

Bonus: Solutions that will keep you sticking to your diet

Staying committed to a diet can be challenging, but implementing these strategies can help you remain focused and motivated:

1. **Meal Planning:**
   - Arrange your meals and snacks ahead of time to guarantee you always have wholesome selections on hand.

2. **Variety in Recipes:**

o   Explore diverse and flavorful recipes within the constraints of your diet to prevent monotony and enhance satisfaction.

3. **Stocking Kidney-Friendly Foods:**

   o   Keep your pantry and refrigerator stocked with kidney-friendly foods to make adhering to your diet more convenient.

4. **Regular Monitoring:**

   o   Regularly track your progress and dietary choices. This self-awareness

can reinforce positive
behaviors.

5. **Consultation with Healthcare Professionals:**

   - Seek guidance from healthcare professionals or dietitians who can provide personalized advice and address any concerns.

6. **Support System:**

   - Share your dietary goals with friends or family who can provide encouragement and accountability.

7. **Gradual Changes:**

   - Implement dietary changes gradually to allow for easier

adaptation and reduce the
likelihood of feeling
overwhelmed.

8. Mindful Eating:

- Practice mindful eating by
  savoring each bite, paying
  attention to hunger and
  fullness cues, and avoiding
  distractions during meals.

9. Educational Resources:

- Utilize educational resources
  to learn more about your
  specific dietary requirements
  and explore new recipes that
  align with your needs.

10.   Positive Reinforcement:

- Celebrate small victories and milestones in your dietary journey to maintain a positive mindset.

Remember that maintaining a healthy diet is a lifestyle change, and it's essential to be patient with yourself. Consistency over time is key, and building habits gradually can lead to long-term success. If you encounter challenges, don't hesitate to seek professional guidance for personalized support.

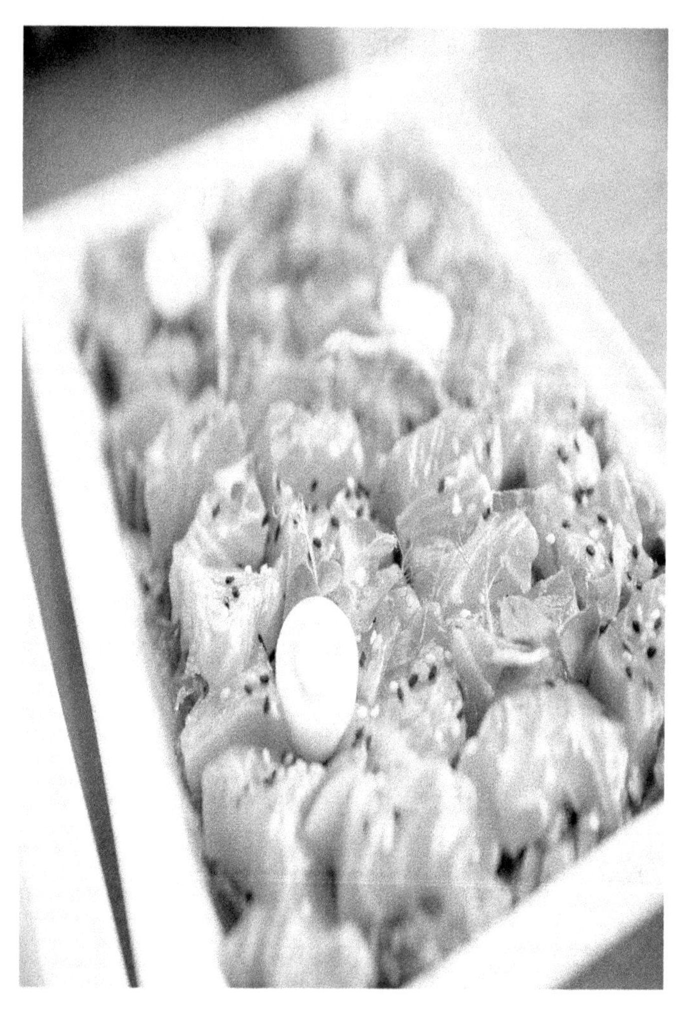

Chapter ten

Meal plan:

Certainly! Here's a sample 30-day meal plan for a renal diet cookbook designed for beginners. Keep in mind that individual dietary needs may vary, so it's important to consult with a healthcare professional or dietitian for personalized advice.

Day 1:

- Breakfast: Quinoa Breakfast Bowl with Berries
- Lunch: Grilled Chicken Salad with Mixed Greens

- Snack: Greek Yogurt with Sliced Peaches

- Dinner: Baked Lemon Herb Chicken with Roasted Sweet Potatoes and Green Beans

Day 2:

- Breakfast: Vegetable Omelet with Spinach and Tomatoes

- Lunch: Lentil Soup with Whole-Grain Roll

- Snack: Hummus with Veggie Sticks

- Dinner: Shrimp and Vegetable Skewers with Quinoa

Day 3:

- Breakfast: Greek Yogurt Parfait with Low-Potassium Granola
- Lunch: Chickpea and Spinach Curry over Basmati Rice
- Snack: Fresh Fruit Salad
- Dinner: Mushroom and Spinach Stuffed Peppers with Brown Rice

Day 4:

- Breakfast: Avocado Toast on Whole Grain Bread
- Lunch: Turkey and Vegetable Wrap with Mixed Greens

- Snack: Hard-Boiled Eggs with a Pinch of Salt

- Dinner: Baked Cod with Herb Crust and Roasted Brussels Sprouts

Day 5:

- Breakfast: Millet Porridge with Cinnamon and Sliced Strawberries

- Lunch: Vegetable and Lentil Stew

- Snack: Nuts and Seeds Mix

- Dinner: Eggplant Parmesan with Whole-Grain Pasta

Repeat and modify the plan as needed for the next few days. Adjust portion sizes based on individual dietary restrictions and consult with healthcare professionals for personalized advice. This plan provides variety and emphasizes whole, kidney-friendly foods while limiting phosphorus and sodium intake.

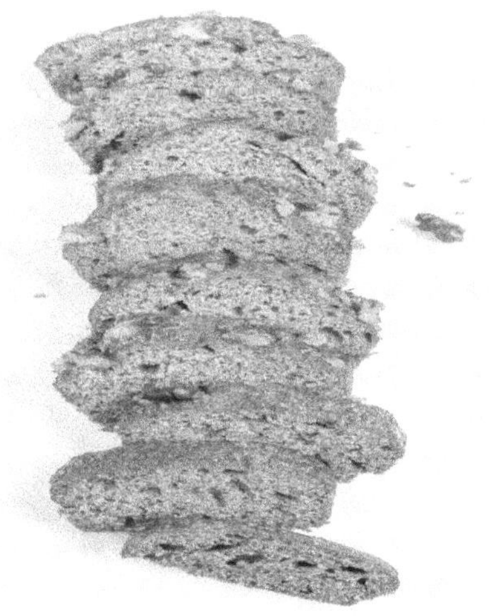

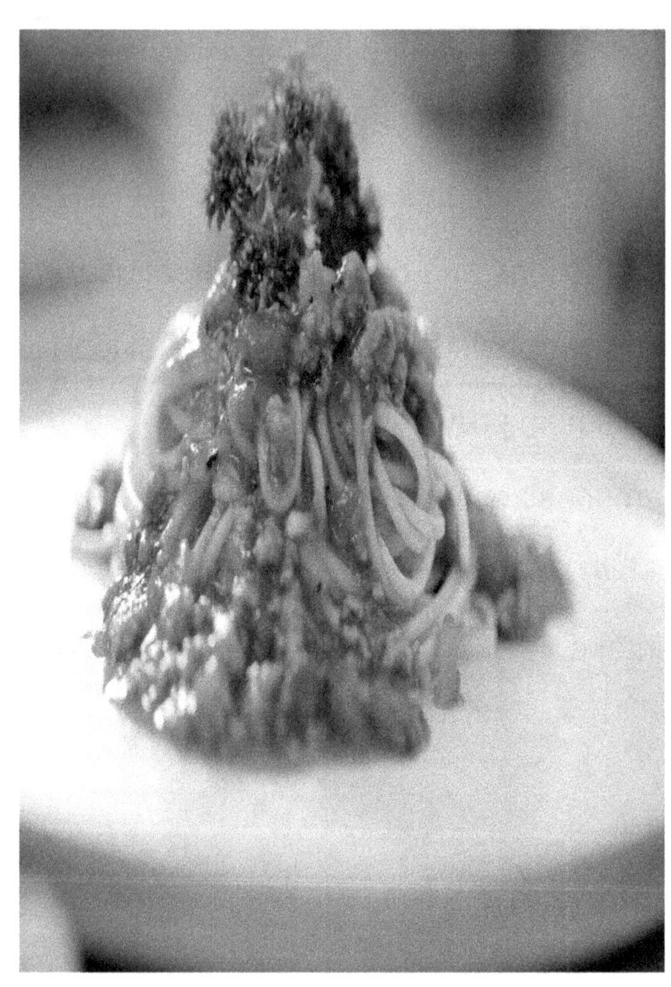

Conclusion

In conclusion, a renal diet cookbook for beginners serves as an invaluable resource in navigating the complexities of a kidney-friendly lifestyle. By offering a diverse array of nutritious recipes, it empowers individuals to embrace a diet tailored to their unique needs. The cookbook not only introduces delicious meals but also cultivates an understanding of how to make informed food choices while managing phosphorus and sodium intake.

Through the careful curation of recipes, this cookbook encourages a positive relationship with food, dispelling the notion that a renal diet must be bland or restrictive. It empowers beginners to explore new flavors, experiment with kidney-friendly ingredients, and discover the pleasure of maintaining a healthy balance.

Furthermore, the cookbook's emphasis on education provides essential insights into the principles of a renal diet, enabling individuals to make informed decisions about their nutrition. As beginners embark on this culinary journey, the cookbook serves as a trusted guide, offering support, inspiration, and practical tips for sustained success.

Ultimately, a renal diet cookbook for beginners not only contributes to the well-being of those with kidney health concerns but also fosters a holistic approach to a healthier lifestyle. By promoting delicious, kidney-friendly meals, it becomes an essential companion on the path to improved health, allowing individuals to savor each bite while prioritizing their well-being.